ONE TO ONE

A Report on Your New Career:
A Retired Nurse Speaks to a New Nurse

ONE TO ONE

A Report on Your New Career:
A Retired Nurse Speaks to a New Nurse

Frances Davis, RN
Three Twenty Publications

DEDICATION

-To Ashlee, my "work-bestie" and the best nurse I have ever known. She is the consummate "Super-Nurse." She is intelligent, kind, encouraging, and thoughtful. She exhibits all the characteristics I describe in this book and more. Her nursing skills are unparalleled, causing all the physicians to love and respect her. Her interpersonal skills cause her patients and her co-workers to love her. Ashlee inspires and sets a wonderful example for us all. And with each shift we share, she inspires and teaches me.

-To Ms. Hall, the very first Super-Nurse I encountered (even though that phrase was not to become popular until decades later.) Her wisdom, nursing skills, and practical knowledge of obstetrics were a gift to so many who worked with her. If you were willing to learn, she would be glad to teach.

-To "Crazy Jess" (her choice of names, not mine). Always moving fast, ponytail swinging behind her, Jess impresses me whenever I observe her excellent nursing care. I tell her often that I want to be like her "when I grow up."

-This dedication is especially to my husband, Glen. Without him, I would never have become the nurse I am. He is my source of strength and encouragement. He has made my life as a nurse infinitely easier over the last 45 years. He has guarded my sleep, ensured I ate enough, and that my scrubs were clean. He has supported me, encouraged me, comforted me, and strengthened me through every single shift. I could not have made 45 years without him.

Frannie and Ashlee

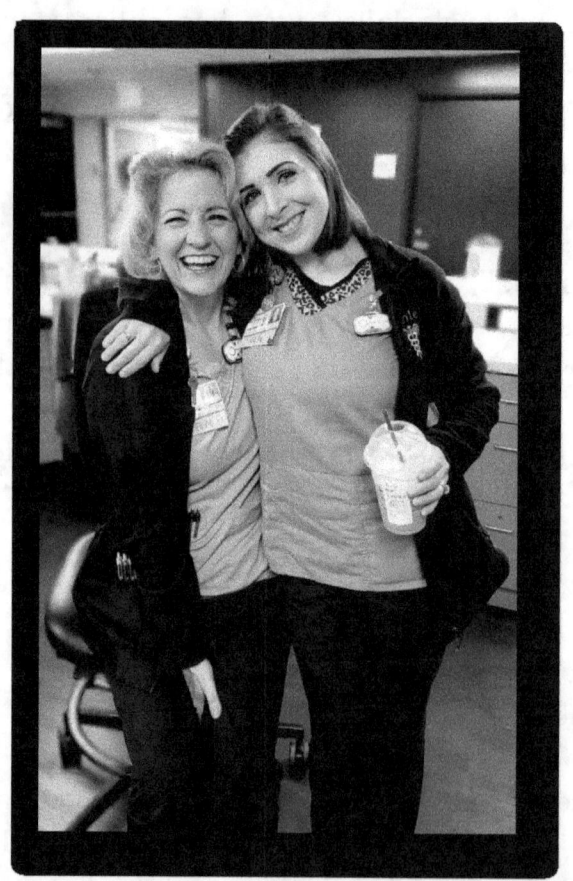

Table of Contents

INTRODUCTION

If you are reading this book, you are a new nurse or about to be a new nurse. Congratulations on your accomplishment!

Graduating from a nursing program is a challenging and incredible achievement. Of course, new nurses also must pass the NCLEX. If you have already sailed over that hurdle, welcome to the family of nurses. It is a wonderful family and a wonderful profession. You will bond with your co-workers in ways you would have never imagined. Sharing the solemn task of protecting life brings together nurses from all backgrounds and lifestyles, sharing a love for what we have chosen to do. Our profession is one in which people will remember us for the rest of their lives. We touch more hearts than we can imagine, and our hearts are touched in return.

Most nurses are familiar with the phrase "one-to-one." It denotes a patient with a complicated condition. They need a nurse who only cares for them. Most new nurses are not up to this task, nor should they be expected to provide that level of care yet. That time will come.

With every one-to-one patient, there is a one-to-one report. This book is much like that shift report, with one retired nurse giving the new nurse the pertinent information on the patient. Except "the patient" is your new career. You will need to tend to it, care for it, and enable it to thrive just as you do your patients.

You may have been asked, "What type of nurse do you want to be?" I ask you that also. My question is, do you want to be a mediocre nurse, a good nurse, a great nurse, or the best nurse possible? What type of nurse you become is entirely up to you.

I have observed the whole continuum of nursing behaviors in my career. The best nurses have characteristics that make them stand out from their peers. I want to share some of these characteristics with you in hopes they will help you along your nursing journey. May that journey lead you to become the best nurse you can be.

The advice I offer in this book is from my own career experiences. It represents things I wish someone had told me when I stepped into a Nurse's Station as an RN for the very first time.

Though my stories are all L&D related, the truths apply to nurses of all specialties.

ONE

HONE YOUR CRAFT

It is only by doing the skill repeatedly that we become skillful.

One hallmark of every outstanding nurse is the execution of nursing skills. She is the person everyone calls for help. She will be the go-to person for IVs. She will have an excellent ear for breath, bowel, and heart sounds. She can put a catheter in anyone! Outstanding OB nurses will be accurate with cervical exams.

It is common to feel inadequate with your skills when first working as a nurse. There is a cure for that. If you are still in your nursing program, ask a professor for instruction. If a simulation lab is available to you, take advantage of it. During your practicum, perform as many skills and as many different types of skills as possible.

If you are already a nurse, ask if you can start all the IVs on your shift. Or put in all the catheters. Whatever your weak area is, *embrace it!* So often, feeling inadequate in a skill makes us want to avoid it. We must overcome that feeling and seek out opportunities to improve. Try to get as much practice as you can. It is only by doing the skill repeatedly that we become skillful. If you work in a hospital, ask if you can spend some mornings in Pre-op just starting IVs. Speak to the nurses in the Education Department and see if you can spend some time in the Skills Lab if your institution has one. Work on your skills so you feel more confident. You will find needing assistance from others becomes a rare occurrence.

Once, I was the Assistant Nurse Manager of our Labor & Delivery unit and oversaw our orientation program. We had two nurses on orientation who were excellent at seeking learning opportunities. One day when the census was low, I was planning to go over emergency scenarios with them and was surprised I couldn't find them.

Finally, I found them in our operating room. They had made a "dummy" patient out of packets of supplies. They were dressed in sterile gowns and gloves and had draped their "patient." They had the education book open to the section on scrubbing in a Caesarean Section. They were practicing, each taking turns, one being the surgeon and the other being the scrub nurse. I was very impressed.

One of the two left us shortly after her orientation. The other became the best nurse I have ever seen.

You will never regret searching out ways to improve your skills.

TWO

CARING ABOUT,

NOT JUST FOR

Being an outstanding nurse is as much about the heart as the mind.

For a large part of my career, my most important role to my patients was that of the teacher. I wanted my patients to understand why we were doing what we did, how we were doing it, what was happening in their bodies, and what was happening with their babies. This education was fine, but I missed the main point.

One patient sent the nurses a "Thank You" card after discharge. In it, she described specific reasons for expressing appreciation to each nurse. She thanked me for "being so informative." While I appreciated her thoughtfulness, the card left me disappointed. Not in her, but in myself for not having had a more personal impact on her.

Eventually, I realized what my patients wanted and needed was for me to care about them. Not just care *for* them but *about* them. Caring for them wasn't meant to be checking off boxes on a to-do list. It was to be seeing each patient first as a person. Being an outstanding nurse is as much about the heart as the mind. We must be able to not only give excellent nursing care but to do it in a way the patient feels we have nothing to do but meet their needs. Of course, that is far from the truth. Every moment we spend with a patient, a part of our brain reminds us of everything else we need to be doing that very second.

We must master the unhurried appearance, which can be difficult during many shifts. Sitting down is one of the best ways to present an air of patience. Patients perceive you have spent much more time with them if you are sitting. They are also more likely to ask questions. We may find we listen to our patients better when sitting as well.

Our goal should be to care for our patients in a way that they feel cared about, not just cared for.

THREE

BE PREPARED

Being prepared isn't paranoia. It is good nursing care.

It is always better to prepare ahead of time for emergencies, admissions, procedures, and anything that affects our patients. Preparing a room before admitting a patient helps the process be as seamless as possible and shows the patient they are cared for by a professional, competent team. While this may not always be possible, our goal should be for this to be the rule rather than the exception.

I noticed a nurse from a different unit admitting a patient recently. She had brought everything she needed with her. She didn't have to interrupt the admitting process, making it much smoother for her and the patient.

A nurse must be prepared for anything and should never have the attitude, "That won't happen in my unit." Even in Labor & Delivery, patients can code. Babies can code, as well. We must check that all the emergency equipment is nearby for any unexpected situation.

Take a few seconds in each patient's room to look around. What equipment might be missing? What possible fall risks are present? Can the furniture be adjusted better for this patient? Is something not functioning that needs to be repaired or replaced? Is there something blocking access to emergency equipment?

Over forty years ago, when I was a new Labor & Delivery nurse, I was shocked one night when one of our patients coded. She had experienced a rare obstetrical emergency. The code team in the delivery room called out for a defibrillator. I didn't know where to find our defibrillator or even if we had one. We *did* have one, but it took valuable minutes for me to find it.

It is much better to have everything you may need close and not need it than to need it and wait for someone to bring it to you. Those seconds, or minutes, can be critical to our patient's outcome.

Being prepared isn't paranoia. It is good nursing care. Our patients expect this of us.

FOUR

DEALING WITH
EMERGENCIES

We may still feel the fear, but we do not act on it.

Knowing we will face emergencies leads to some degree of fear as nurses. Fear can be a good thing. It keeps us alert and watchful. Emergencies are real challenges with possible detrimental consequences. The fear of emergencies is a challenge won first in our heads before we ever face it in our units.

When I first started in Labor & Delivery, three things frightened me. One was a seizing patient. The second was being the scrub nurse on an emergency Cesarean Section. The third was a hemorrhaging patient. What frightened me most, however, was finding myself in an emergency and not knowing what to do.

To be ready for those situations, I memorized the steps of what to do. Then I visualized the scenario and pictured myself taking the appropriate steps in the proper order.

It didn't take long for me to encounter the situations I feared. The study and visualization paid off. Even though I still felt fear, I responded appropriately in those situations. I replaced those first three fears with more things and then more again. Finally, I had encountered most of the things I feared and some things I hadn't even known to fear.

Emergencies are real. They will eventually happen to each one of us. We must ensure we know what to do and have the skills to match our knowledge.

The urge to scream or cry in an emergency is normal. New nurses tend to freeze with fear in these situations. We must learn to push our feelings to the back of our minds. We will function quickly and efficiently if we are mentally prepared. We may still feel the fear, but we do not act on it. We implement the policies and protocols we have learned through the skills we have mastered. Later, we deal with our emotions.

One day, a physician brought over a patient with low fetal heart tones for an emergency Cesarean Section.

I had a nurse on orientation with me, and I told her to stand still and watch. Two shifts of nurses were in the operating room preparing the patient, the surgical equipment, and the baby's emergency equipment and assisting anesthesia personnel.

No one said anything during that time. Each nurse just looked at what had been done and what was being done. Then, they found something that *needed* to be done. It was like a beautiful nursing ballet. There was no confusion, raised voices, or apparent fear (although I'm sure we all felt it.) Within a few minutes, the baby was born and did very well.

That birth happened as it did because each nurse knew the essential processes. They knew what to do and in which order things were to be done.

Their knowledge was one of the things that made the difference between a baby that did well and one that didn't.

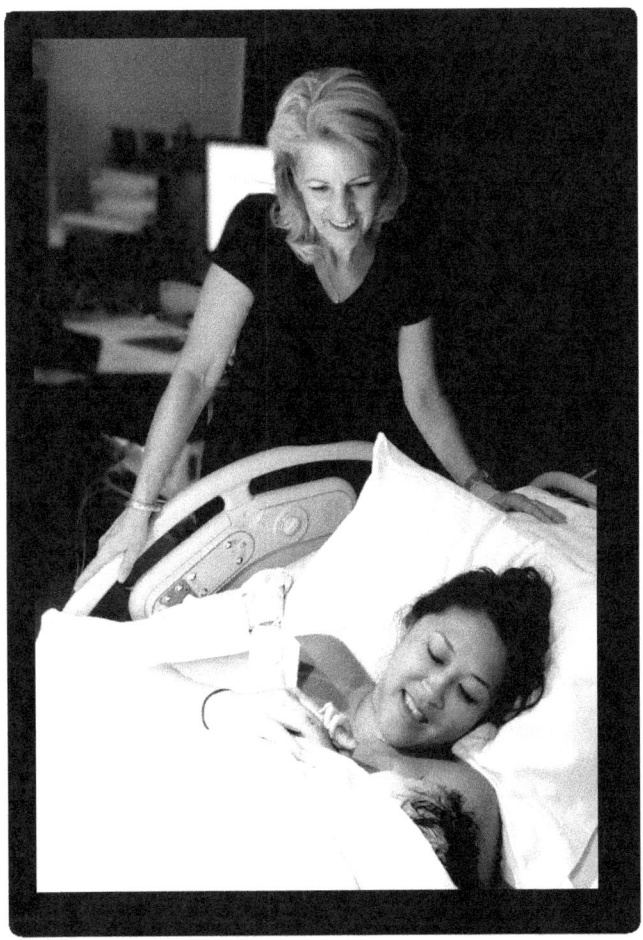

FIVE

NEVER ASSUME THE BEST

Always investigate the abnormal findings on your patient.

Some nurses assume that everything is wrong until it is proven right, and some think everything is right until it is proven wrong.

Sometimes, our patient can have abnormal vital signs or lab results and still be okay. But to believe that without substantiation is poor nursing practice. There is always the possibility things are *not* okay. Abnormal lab results, vital signs, etc., should lead us to assess further, implement interventions, and reassess. This is the heart of the nursing process and is the nursing care plan in action.

Suppose our patient has elevated blood pressure. We may justify the elevation, thinking the patient is in pain or whatever rationale we believe caused the abnormal blood pressure. That may be true, but we need to substantiate that. Did the blood pressure go down after we gave the patient pain medication? The patient's pain and hypertension may be different but concurrent problems.

We should assess abnormal vital signs as just that and react accordingly. If the patient is fine, and we do what we know to do, everything will likely continue to be fine. If the patient truly is hypertensive (or whatever the issue is) to the degree intervention is necessary - and we don't intervene - our patient may experience a bad outcome.

By investigating abnormal results on our patients and actively intervening, when necessary, we have the best hope of our patients having good outcomes.

Once, I had a patient on a continuous Magnesium drip. Protocols for a Magnesium drip for pre-eclampsia called for blood pressure, deep tendon reflexes, and assessment of urine output every hour.

The patient had a slightly low blood pressure (which can occur from the effects of the Magnesium). Her urine output was also slightly decreased. Neither of these were too concerning. When I spoke to her, she told me she was very fatigued. When I checked her deep tendon reflexes, I knew why. She had no reflexes, which can be a sign of Magnesium toxicity. I turned the Magnesium drip off and immediately drew a STAT Magnesium level. The level was almost 50% higher than the top range of therapeutic. I notified the physician, and the Magnesium was not resumed. The patient continued without further consequence. She could have coded if I assumed she was "really okay" and not assessed further. Standards of Care and Policies and Protocols are in place to protect our patients. It is expected of us to follow them.

Always investigate the abnormal findings on your patient.

SIX

ASK FOR HELP

When we work as a team, everything goes so much smoother.

I once heard, "Asking for help when you need it is not an admission of weakness. It is an expression of maturity."

We *all* need help from time to time. Never hesitate to ask for help. If you ask for help, the other nurses will understand. It is much better to ask for help and have the patient's needs met promptly than to struggle on our own and make our patient wait needlessly. At some point, it will be your turn to return the favor.

Simply asking for help from one nurse is one thing, but sometimes, we need more than one person to help. Don't hesitate to pull the call light out of the wall in an emergency. Usually, this gets a quick response from multiple staff members. Some hospitals have implemented "Staff Emergency" buttons into the call light system. If this is available, use it when necessary. When needed, call a Rapid Response.

Once, I received a patient from the ER. She was bleeding more profusely than I had ever seen in my life. I didn't want to frighten the patient, so I put on the call light and told the nurse, who answered, "I'm going to need some help here."

When the nurse came into the room and saw all the blood on the floor, she knew we needed even more help. Had I just pulled the cord from the wall or used the "Staff Emergency" button, several staff members would have been in my room in seconds.

Sometimes, it's just the best thing to do.

SEVEN

GIVE HELP

Asking if someone needs help is not the same as helping.

Knowing how it feels to need help is why we should be quick to *give help*.

It doesn't help a coworker to ask if she needs help after she has finally finished catching up. Asking if someone needs help is not the same as helping.

If a co-worker is struggling during the shift, we should not only ask if there is anything we can do for them. We should do whatever we *know* needs to be done. If one of their patients calls out for something and it is within our power to help them, we should do so. The nurse, 99 times out of 100, will be so grateful for the help.

As a new nurse, you may feel there is little you can offer to help, however even the easiest thing is one less thing our co-worker must do. Anything we can take their patient is one less thing they must get and take to the room. Many little things can add up to a big thing.

Sometimes, listening out for their other patients is the most significant help we can give our co-workers. Giving help will almost always come back to you multiplied.

It was only a short time after I went PRN (working only two shifts a month) I realized I could go weeks or months between performing some procedures.

I had a laboring patient one shift that needed a C-Section. I couldn't believe it had been ten months since I had circulated on a C-Section! Fortunately, when I called out to the nurses' station for Anesthesia, my charge nurse realized what was happening and came into my room with her arms full of the things I would need to pre-op my patient and take her to the OR. Her help was invaluable to me.

If it is within your power to do so, always try to help your co-workers. It is part of being the best nurse you can be.

Many years ago, two Labor & Delivery nurses in our unit started helping other nurses in extraordinary ways. They prepared the patient's room for delivery. They helped while the patient was pushing and during the delivery. After delivery, they did everything they could to help the nurse catch up. Other nurses who had received this help sought opportunities to help others.

These nurses created an atmosphere of support and teamwork through their actions. The patient's nurse didn't have to ask for help; it just appeared. The nurses all worked together as a team, and when a team completes work, everything goes so much smoother. The patients usually feel more secure and cared for, and nurses' attitudes improve.

EIGHT

CALL THE DOCTOR

You are not there to be the physician's friend; you are there to take care of your patient.

New nurses are often very hesitant to call the physician, especially in the middle of the night. I have reassured many new nurses that they must call the physician even though the doctor may be unhappy. I have also reassured them the physician will get over it. I have told them that no one has ever been named in a lawsuit because they called the doctor. Some have been, however, because they did not.

I often recommend new nurses write down what they want to say to the doctor. Include all the pertinent information but leave out the things unimportant to the issue. If you feel comfortable, practice what to report to the physician with another nurse. A more experienced nurse will often be glad to sit with you while you call the physician until you get comfortable calling them. Before you know it, you will be the nurse reassuring a newer one!

When calling a physician in the middle of the night, make sure you are calling the correct physician. Verify which physician is on call for that group or service. Verify you have the correct physician and the right patient. Those two steps will go a long way to keep you from dealing with an irritated physician in the middle of the night.

If you call the doctor and they are rude, if they yell at you, or are unprofessional in any way, ignore it. You are not there to be the physician's friend but to care for your patient.

Write down what the doctor says to you as they give you orders. Don't trust your memory. You will regret it if you call them back to repeat it. Then, read the orders back to them. *Do not skip this step!*

If the orders seem unusual or inconsistent with the expected plan of care, question the orders.

One night in 1978, I was fresh out of my nursing program, and a doctor left a full sheet of written orders on his new admission. His handwriting was absolutely atrocious. A more experienced nurse and I deciphered those orders until we reached the last one. It was only one word, but neither of us could figure it out. By then it was 3:00 a.m., and the other nurse told me I had to call him. I didn't want to, but I did. Quite curtly, he told me the last order was "Thanks." We were both frustrated that we had spent so much time and energy on deciphering his last "order." I am glad we didn't ignore it though, because it could actually have been something crucial to the patient's care.

Be aware that some people can have perfectly cogent conversations while asleep. I have known several physicians like this. Usually, after calling them about a patient in the middle of the night, they will call back and ask, "What did I tell you to do about that patient?" The orders they give while awake may differ from those they give in sleep.

If you are concerned a patient's condition is deteriorating, *be clear about it*. Tell them that directly. Don't hope they read between the lines or take your hint. If you want them to come and see the patient, clearly tell them; don't be vague. If they refuse to come to assess the patient, activate your chain of command.

Once, we had a patient with a fetal heart rate tracing that none of us were comfortable with. It wasn't bad at that point, but it wasn't reassuring, either. The physician, who lived close to the hospital, wanted to go home briefly. I told the physician I was uncomfortable with his choice and concerned about his leaving the hospital. I also told him I was very uneasy with the fetal monitoring tracing. I told him these things not only to convey my concern but also so I could chart what I had told him. *I told him that as well.*

If you call a physician, chart it. In any unusual situation, I prefer to quote what I said and the physician's response in the patient's chart.

Calling a physician, especially at night, is never fun. But it is a necessary part of the job.

If you have that nagging feeling you should call the doctor, do it, get it over with, and *always* chart it.

NINE

BE QUICK TO PRAISE

Take every opportunity to say something kind, uplifting or encouraging to others.

We all like to hear we did a good job. We each have the power to make others feel good about the job they have done. We underestimate how our positive comments can encourage, strengthen, and comfort those around us. You may think your praise wouldn't mean much because you are a new nurse, but that is not true. As well as making the recipient of your thoughtfulness feel good, it shows you are a kind and caring person.

During my first five years as a nurse, I worked in the NICU. One day, I was standing at one of my babies' warmers, and my co-worker called my name. When I looked up, she said, "I like you."

That was it, just those three words. It may have been a small sentence, but it made a big impression, especially since it came from an experienced nurse I respected and liked.

Take every opportunity to say something kind, uplifting, or encouraging to others. You may never know how that one comment can ignite a fire of confidence inside someone. It may give them strength they didn't have before.

Better yet, write a note. Notes are tangible evidence of what a person is feeling at the time. They can be read and reread. It can be as heart-warming over time as it was when first read.

Better still is a letter to that nurse's manager. Let someone know if that person has performed in a way that truly impressed you.

If someone points out your great job with a patient, remember to mention the care tech, secretary, or other nurses who helped you.

When watching football, I hate to see the receiver make a show of himself in the end zone about his touchdown. Did he forget the front line that kept the other team from running over him? A team is a group of people working toward a common goal. Nursing performed as a team is always better.

Recognize and thank your team whenever you can.

You never know what seed for the future may be planted by your thoughtful words and actions.

TEN

GUARD YOUR TONGUE

Treat people with respect, even if they disrespect you.
Do so because of who you are.

Sometimes, you will have the perfect comeback, the smartest, sharpest remark on the tip of your tongue. It needs to stay there.

Whoever is the target of your words, your patient, their family, a co-worker, or a physician, there is no place for unprofessional behavior from a nurse.

Once released, words can return to haunt us when we least expect it. We can avoid much trouble by guarding our tongues.

Our opinion is rarely essential to the performance of our jobs. Respecting our patients, their families, our co-workers, and the physicians is paramount. We can never be sure who is listening to, watching, or even videoing us. Sometimes, we may drop the professional attitude at the nurses' station and chat with friends. When we do, usually, at least some of our patients can hear the nurses' station from their rooms. Visitors and other staff members walk by all the time. It is better to maintain our professionalism all the time and save the rest for socializing away from your job.

During a nursing career, we will encounter and care for people from all walks of life, with many different life experiences, preferences, and choices. They all deserve our respect.

Once, I was the circulating nurse in a Cesarean Section, and the surgeon was rude to the scrub nurse. She continued her job calmly and politely, ignoring his tirade. Her "Yes, sir" and "No, sir" were a contrast to the rude things he was calling all of us. After the surgery, I spoke to her about it.

"Connie," I asked, "How could you treat him so politely when he was being such a jerk?"

She replied with one of the most profound answers I have heard.

"I don't treat him politely because of who he is or what he does," she said. "I treat him that way because of who *I am*."

That moment was a great life lesson.

Treat people with respect, even if they disrespect you. Do so because of who *you* are.

ELEVEN

LEARN FROM EVERYONE

Everyone brings strengths, knowledge, and skills others can learn and utilize.

Look for opportunities to learn, they are everywhere. Every single housekeeper, technician, phlebotomist, physician, nurse, visitor, and patient can teach us something.

I had been a Labor & Delivery nurse for many years when "Obstetric Scrub Technicians" came into our unit. They were responsible for setting up sterile tables for surgeries. While each setup had the same number and type of instruments, each scrub technician set their tables up a little differently, and I enjoyed looking at the different setups. One tech set up her Cesarean Section table unlike any other I had seen. But when I watched her during the surgery, I realized it was also the most efficient setup I had ever seen. I started setting my tables up that way and have been doing so for over twenty years.

Recently, I was in a delivery with a much younger nurse. The way she coached and encouraged the patient was perfect. Not only what she said but *how* she said it. I am determined to remember the way she gave positive encouragement to the patient the next time I was in that position.

Everyone brings strengths, knowledge, and skills others can learn and utilize.

You will not only learn by watching, but by asking as well. Don't hesitate to get a second opinion from another nurse. Sometimes, it is easy to overlook the obvious. Ask for their opinion if you struggle with a particular skill or situation. You may be missing what you need to say or do.

When on the Mother-Baby unit, I often consult the most experienced Nursery nurse for insights and expertise when faced with an unfamiliar situation. In that instance, you can chart that you did so. It shows you sought out advice and assistance.

The nurse who does not realize she can learn from other staff members has the most to learn from everyone.

Once, a nurse was helping me admit a patient. She was going to put the patient on the fetal monitor, but first, she asked, "Do you mind if I pull up your gown a bit to put you on the monitor?"

I remember thinking at the time how thoughtful that was and how I had never heard anyone ask that before. This Super-Nurse knew that some patients may have a history of abuse, which may make being uncovered without consent an uncomfortable event. Her simple act spoke much of her care and concern for the patient. Without even trying, she taught me how to be a better nurse.

TWELVE

"IT IS YOUR JOB AND EVERYONE'S JOB UNDERNEATH YOU!"

As nurses, there is nothing in the care of a patient that is beneath us.

One night, when I was new to Labor & Delivery, we were swamped and needed a Delivery Room cleaned. Housekeeping was not available. The Charge Nurse told me to come with her to clean the Delivery Room.

Young and too full of myself, I answered, "That's not in my job description!"

Gently, but seriously, she replied, "Your job description is your job and every job underneath you! Now, here's your mop!"

She was not one to be challenged. She knew more about Labor and Delivery in her sleep than I did on my best day. Together, we cleaned the room.

I have quoted her many times in my career. As nurses, nothing in the care of a patient is beneath us. Does the patient need her trash taken out? Yes, we can do that. Does the floor need to be swept? Yes, we can do that, too. Does she need help with breastfeeding? Yes, we can help. Does she want some juice and crackers? Yes, we can take that to her.

We can and should delegate appropriate tasks to ancillary staff when possible. However, the patient should not wait to receive what they need if we can provide it.

One night about midnight, I finished assessing a postpartum patient and she asked if I could call Housekeeping to clean her floor. She told me her husband had dropped his bottle of soda on the floor and now the floor was sticky.

I explained to her that I would be back in a minute to clean her floor. She said she didn't want me to do it, she just wanted Housekeeping to know. I knew that nightshift Housekeeping was stretched tightly between ER, OR, and L&D and it was unlikely her floor would be cleaned before morning.

I came back with a mop and broom and as I turned on the light the patient said, "Oh, I should tell you that bottle was glass."

Indeed, there was broken glass all over the floor. As I got on my hands and knees to make sure I had all the broken shards, I noticed broken glass was even in her slippers at the bedside.

I was so glad the patient had not put her slippers on to get out of bed. Her feet could have been badly cut.

I had intended to clean the floor anyway but seeing that made me glad that I had.

THIRTEEN

NURSES NEED TO HEAL, TOO

Try to remember to care for yourself as if you were caring for your patients.

On the very best of shifts, nursing is hard. Add a few under-staffed shifts, a couple of complicated patients, and an impatient physician, and it can be exhausting.

When we finish our shifts and go home, most likely we don't sleep enough or well enough. We are often too tired to exercise or to socialize with friends. We carry stress from our jobs even when we are away from the workplace.

Try to remember to care for yourself as if you were caring for your patients. Eat well. Eat *enough*. Drink more water. Rest when you are tired. Find time to do things you enjoy, even if only sitting outside watching the clouds pass by.

Limit the times you work extra when the unit calls for help. While your co-workers greatly appreciate it when you work extra, your body and mind will not. It is beneficial for you to have time away from the workplace. Nursing is stressful, not just on our minds and emotions, but on our necks, backs, and legs. Give yourself time to heal.

Remember to take vacations! Time away is a great healer. Do something that makes you laugh and smile. Enjoy the things you love and the people you love. You will return to work refreshed, recharged, and ready to give all you are to your patients.

Part of healing yourself is to take care of yourself in the first place. Don't make yourself the last priority. Sometimes, it isn't possible, but take your lunch break during your shift when you can. Go to the bathroom when you need to. A gynecologist once told me that nurses and teachers always had bigger bladders than other women. He thought it was because we often couldn't go to the bathroom when we first felt the need. If you need to go, GO!

Protect your legs by wearing compression socks. Use proper body mechanics when moving patients.

If you are sick, stay home and get well. You deserve to rest when you are ill, and your co-workers will be glad you didn't share whatever you have with them.

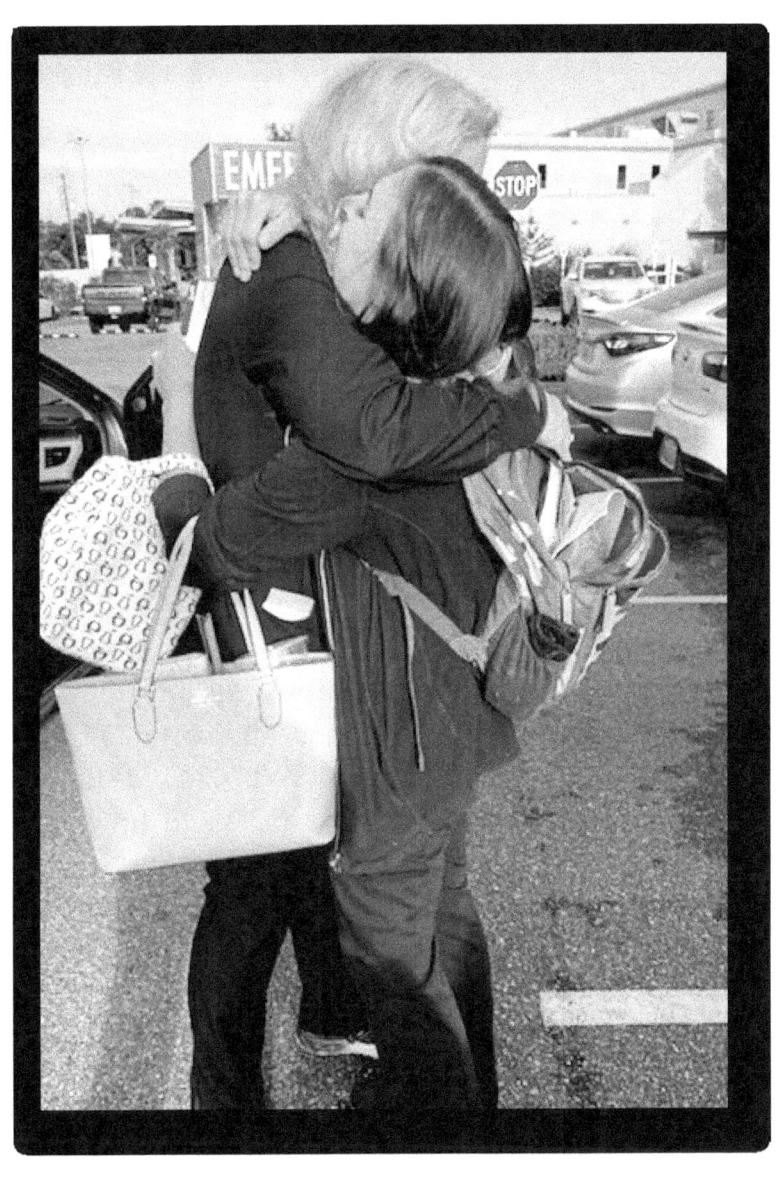

Nurses help each other heal, too.

FOURTEEN

WATCH OTHER NURSES

Most experienced nurses enjoy sharing their knowledge with new nurses, especially when they see you are willing to learn.

Watch what other nurses do and how they do it. Listen to how they talk with the patients, the questions they ask, and how they phrase the admission questions. Watch how they perform their nursing skills. Observe how they start IVs and how they put in Foley catheters. Listen to how they give report and how they discuss the patient with physicians. Most experienced nurses enjoy sharing their knowledge with new nurses, especially when they see you are willing to learn.

One nurse, not long out of orientation, was taking advantage of our low census to ask questions regarding emergency procedures. Less than an hour after she asked what to do in case of a fire, the fire alarm for the Postpartum unit went off.

Thinking it was a test, I walked that way. As I turned onto the Postpartum hallway, I saw a Care Technician at the other end of the hall grab the fire extinguisher. My heart began to race, and I ran in the direction of the Care Tech.

I found a hallway full of smoke. We evacuated the Nursery to a pre-designated spot. Labor & Delivery had no patients at the time, so we turned off the oxygen and sent the Labor & Delivery nurses to help the Nursery with the evacuation, and to be ready for anything.

Once the Firefighters arrived, we learned all the smoke was from a faulty ballast in a light bulb.

I was proud that our newest nurse had the foresight to ask questions about the procedures, and shortly –very shortly- thereafter see them in action.

Never be afraid of asking questions.

FIFTEEN

THE PATIENT'S SUPPORT SYSTEM

We cannot project how we want to be treated onto our patients.

You will only have practiced as a nurse briefly before encountering a patient's family member who irritates you. It may be the family nurse who, although she knows nothing about your specialty, wants to tell you how to do your job. Perhaps the patient's grandma constantly wants to prepare the patient for what will happen next. Only her advice needs to be updated. Maybe it is a spouse who wants to make every decision for the patient to the point the patient doesn't even answer when you ask a question.

We may disagree with the patient's support system and even think they hinder our patient care. We may think they should treat our patient with more respect, but we must remember this is our *patient's* support system, not ours. We must also remember they know much more about our patient than we do. We cannot project how *we* want to be treated onto our patients.

Our patient will be going home with these people. If we are rude to the patient's family and friends, or treat them with disrespect, our patient will not appreciate it. They may not accept our teaching or advice, either. We don't want to put the patient in a position to choose between the family or the nurse. If we do, we can be sure the nurse will never win.

We must actively teach the family as we teach the patient and try our best to include them in the discharge plan of care. We must especially validate what they say and do that is helpful to our patient's recovery.

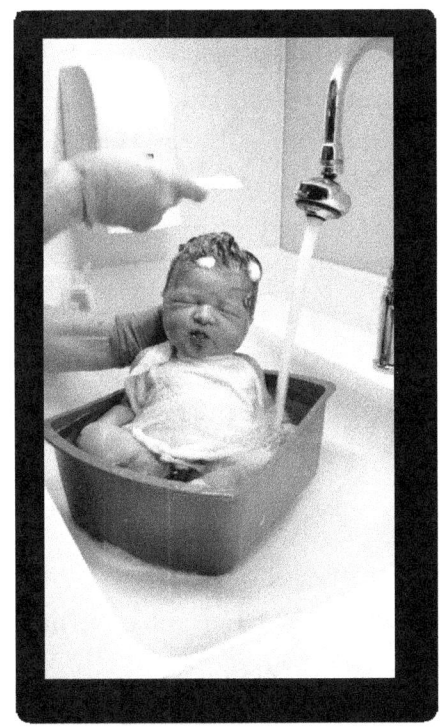

SIXTEEN

SHOUT ONLY WHEN NECESSARY

Use screaming sparingly so when you need to do it, it means something.

Once, I worked with a nurse who shouted *a lot*. She was an excellent nurse, but she screamed as her chief way of getting help. It probably frightened her patient and the patients in the adjoining rooms. I know it frequently scared me!

There are times, however, when screaming for help may be appropriate.

One night in L&D, a mild-mannered intern quietly asked how he could contact the anesthesia personnel.

I was curious and asked, "Scott, why do you need anesthesia?"

"We have a prolapsed cord in room 6," was his calm reply.

I was stunned. A prolapsed cord is an obstetrical emergency requiring a lot of help.

"This is how you do it," I said to him. Then I screamed, "Prolapsed cord in 6!"

Nurses ran from every direction, and in seconds, they rolled the patient past us to the OR.

Scott looked at me, shocked, and said, "Thank you."

Use shouting sparingly so when you need to do it, it means something.

SEVENTEEN

TREAT YOUR NURSE MANAGER WITH RESPECT

Our nurse managers deserve our support and our respect.

As a new nurse, you may not know your Nurse Manager well yet. Take every opportunity you can to get to know them.

I had one nurse manager who was simply non-existent. I worked the night shift, and we never saw her. Weeks would go by without us even hearing from her.

I had one manager who not only knew all the employees in the unit; she knew their spouse's names, their children's names, and sometimes their pets' names! She made a point to speak to each staff member at the beginning of the shift. If she knew someone in your family was ill, she would ask how they were doing. If she ever had to reprimand someone, she did so in the privacy of her office, and she always had some word of praise for them before they left. These acts of respect endeared her to her staff.

I had one nurse manager who was an "in the trenches" type of manager. She wouldn't be in her office with the door closed if the unit was busy. She would be on the unit, taking patients herself and usually taking the heaviest load. She worked elbow to elbow with her staff. This selfless giving of herself to her unit endeared her to them.

Each manager has positive traits and negative traits. Regardless of which they have more of, being a nurse manager is a complex and relentless job. When a manager walks across the parking lot at the end of the day, their job continues. They are most likely thinking about problems that need to be solved, and issues they will have to deal with the following day. They may be wondering how they are going to balance the unit's budget. It is like wearing a heavy coat every moment.

Most managers request to be notified if there is an unusual occurrence or a bad outcome. Some will come to the unit to offer comfort and support to the involved staff.

Our nurse managers deserve our support and our respect. Most staff nurses would only last a short time with the work and responsibility expected of a manager.

If we have a complaint with our Nurse Manager, we should give them the same respect we would want. Ask for an appointment with them to discuss the issue privately. Discussing whatever it is with the rest of the staff only leads to decreased morale and workplace dissatisfaction.

By supporting our managers, we aren't saying we think they are perfect. Instead, it means we support what they do.

Always respect the difficult position your manager willingly takes upon themselves.

EIGHTEEN

NO ONE IS INDISPENSABLE

You cannot make your life decisions based on how they might affect your unit.

At some point in your career, you may want to make a change. It could be to change shifts, units, facilities, or even specialties.

Often, when nurses begin to think these thoughts, they immediately begin to feel guilty. They may think of an already understaffed shift or co-workers who would be left behind. I have always advised someone who wanted to work elsewhere to "Do what is best for you and your family."

You cannot make life decisions based on what will happen in your unit. If you are truly unhappy where you are, and you believe you will be happier somewhere else, you should give it a try. Trust me, the unit will go on. Even tiny units will withstand the loss. Your Nurse Manager will hire another nurse, and life will continue. Nursing is stressful, and you owe it to yourself and your family to be where you believe you will find the most enjoyment and fulfillment.

If you do decide to leave, do so gracefully. Be sure to give notice and work it out. Don't be negative about your current institution to your co-workers. They may not be able to leave as you are. Your statements may lead them to be discontented. Don't be too enthusiastic about your new institution, either. After all, you haven't worked there yet to know what it will be like. Be thoughtful about the co-workers you leave and how it will affect them. Another reason to leave gracefully is because you just may decide you have made a mistake and want to come back. If your exit was pleasant, the door may still be open for you.

Once I had a dear friend who was very frustrated about some changes in our department. She decided to take a position at another hospital in our area. I had worked where she was going for several years and I didn't think it would be a good fit for her, still, I encouraged her to do what she thought was best for herself and her family. Her last day came, and we said our goodbyes. I didn't tell her this, but I was broken-hearted. She was not only a great co-worker, but she was also my best friend. As it turned out, it was *not* a good fit for her, and she quickly realized that. Because she had not burned any bridges when leaving, she was able to cross them again to come back.

But perhaps you will have an experience like mine. I left a stressful, understaffed unit to try another hospital in our town. I don't know why, but when I started at the new hospital, I just felt as if I had "come home." It was much less stressful with ample time to get to know my patients and their families. By the end of my first week, I knew I would never want to work anywhere else.

Nursing can offer great variety throughout a career. If you start in one specialty, you may try another one years later. I have seen Cardiac nurses become L&D Nurses, L&D nurses become Hospice nurses, Nursery nurses become L&D nurses, L&D nurses become Nursery nurses, and hospital nurses become IT nurses. The list could go on and on. You could work in a hospital, a physician's office, or a clinic. You could be a nurse educator or a patient educator. The opportunities almost seem endless. I have worked in the NICU, L&D, IT, Community Education, and Mother-Baby.

If you ever tire of where you are in nursing or find yourself burned out (which does happen), don't be afraid to try something new. You made it through your nursing program and passed the NCLEX; you can learn a new specialty!

Nursing also offers the chance to "see the world," as the old commercial used to say. If you decide to move across the country, you will likely find openings wherever you go. Many nurses take advantage of the benefits offered by travel nursing. I know of one family who packed up an RV and traveled across the United States. While the mom worked as a travel nurse, the dad homeschooled the children, and they visited historic sites in the country in between.

Always make the choice that is best for you and your family.

NINETEEN

KEEP COUNT

Days have a way of blending in your mind, and you won't be able to go back and track the information later.

Over the years, I have kept track of how many deliveries I have been in and roughly how many babies I have delivered myself. But there are so many more things I wish I had counted.

As you go through your shifts, you may want to keep track of things you do. Decades from now, you might find it interesting to know how many IVs you have started or the total number of patients you have cared for. Perhaps you would want to know how many codes you have participated in or how many admissions you have done.

If you like keeping statistics, take a second to jot down your numbers at the end of your shift. Days have a way of blending in your mind, and you won't be able to go back and track the information later. Thirty, forty, or fifty years after starting your nursing career, seeing how much you have accomplished may be interesting.

It will make interesting trivia for your retirement party, too!

Over 4,000 deliveries!

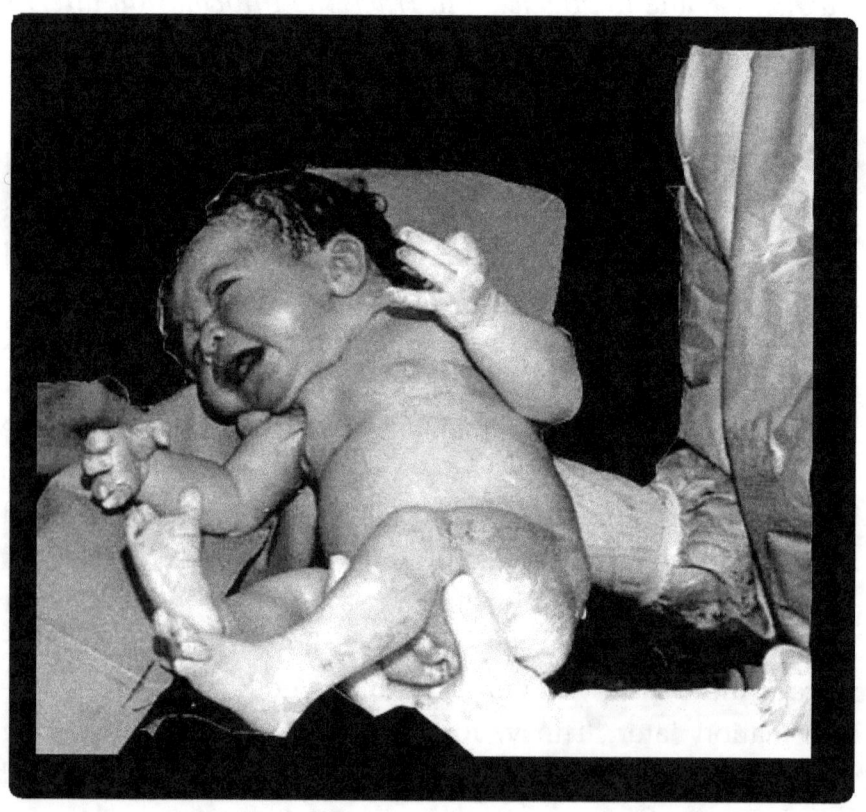

TWENTY

THE NOTEBOOK

It will become a personal reference guide.

Most nurses carry a stethoscope, some have scissors, and a few may carry a hemostat. For a new nurse, I also recommend a small notebook that fits in a pocket.

Especially on orientation, the new nurse can use the notebook to write down anything discussed with the preceptor. The notebook can contain answers to questions, protocols, or drug information. It will become a personal reference guide. You can reread the contents, helping reinforce information previously learned in the unit.

Some new nurses never utilized this tool; others became attached to their notebooks. It gave them a sense of confidence they otherwise lacked.

Denise was one of these nurses. She took on her L&D orientation with passion. She wanted to know *everything*. She had her little notebook with her even long after her orientation ended. (Most who used a notebook did the same.)

One night, we were working together, and she was pulling her things out of her bag: pens, a stethoscope, and scissors, but she couldn't find her notebook.

She wasn't sure she could get through the shift without it, but she did. She stated at the end of the night, "Well, it's the end of the shift, and I didn't miss my notebook. I guess that means I don't need it anymore."

That was precisely what it meant. If you use a notebook as a learning tool, the day will come when you will no longer need it. It will have accomplished its job.

If you hold onto it, one day when you are a preceptor, and can use it as an example to the nurse you are training.

TWENTY-ONE

IT WILL HAPPEN

Body fluid is going to end up on you.

Regardless of how much you try to avoid it, it will happen in your career. Body fluid is going to end up on you.

As disgusting as it is when it happens, there's just not much to do about it at that point. Wash as well as you can, and change clothes when possible.

I was new to Labor & Delivery and was pushing with a woman who had no family with her. Sitting on the side of the bed was the best way for me to help hold her legs while she pushed. From there, I could reach both legs and watch her pushing progress.

Our charge nurse, a wise woman (and a Super-Nurse if there ever was one,) walked past me and softly stated, "I wouldn't do that if I were you."

I turned my head to look at her as she spoke. As I turned back around, my eye noticed something glistening between my patient's legs. Before my mind could comprehend this was her amniotic sac, it burst, and amniotic fluid went everywhere.

It was dripping off my eyelashes and nose. It was running down my chest into my bra. Because I was still sitting on the bed, amniotic fluid covered my whole lap. I could hear the nurses outside the room softly chuckling, probably because they had once been in that position.

I didn't have time to change clothes because the baby was coming right behind the amniotic sac. It was gross then, but now I laugh about my naivety. The best way to avoid contamination with body fluids is to wear the appropriate personal protective equipment. Even then, you may end up with something on you. Sometimes, the best way to deal with gross situations is to laugh. Complaining accomplishes nothing. Laughing at the situation can somehow help it seem not quite so bad.

There is something else that may happen to you as well. You may be the target of a patient's violence, whether intentional or not. Sometimes, patients do not tolerate treatments well and can lash out at the nearest person. In 45 years, patients have twisted my arm, punched, hit, pinched and bitten me.

Once, I was in a tiny labor room to draw blood on a patient, with only about two feet between the bed and the wall. I slipped into this space, explained to the patient the procedure, and proceeded to draw her blood. The moment the needle reached the vein, the patient took her other arm and punched me square in the chest, knocking me against the wall behind me. As I felt my body bounce off the wall, I was surprised to see the tube still in my hand, full of blood!

I was so glad because I knew I wouldn't stick that patient again!

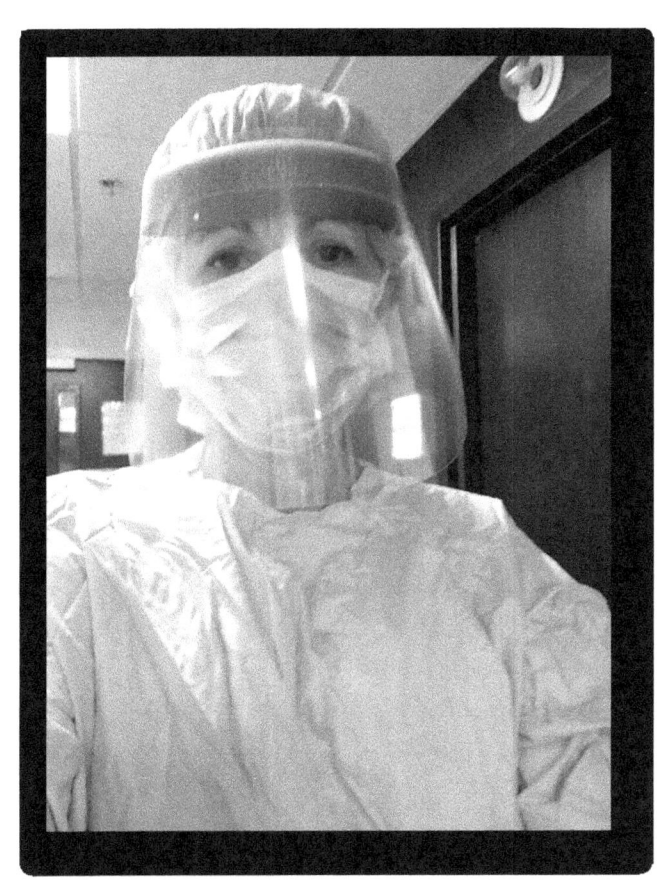

Covid Days

TWENTY-TWO

TAKE RESPONSIBILITY

When we make mistakes, we must take responsibility.

At some point, every nurse will make a mistake. You will feel so disappointed in yourself when this happens, which is normal. When we make mistakes, *we must take responsibility*. Most institutions have a protocol for reporting mistakes or "near-misses." Report your mistake to your Nurse Manager, who can guide you with further steps if necessary. Most Nurse Managers are very understanding, especially if you are reporting your own mistake or near-miss. They have likely been there themselves at some point.

You may not believe it when the mistake occurs, but you will learn a more significant lesson from a mistake than from doing everything perfectly.

I had been in hundreds of deliveries, so inexperience was not an excuse for this mistake. The physician handed me the baby. Part of caring for the baby was to put the plastic umbilical clamp on the umbilical cord and cut away the extra cord. I have done this hundreds of times. But when I went to cut the excess cord off from above the plastic clamp, I cut *below* it instead.

The physician brought me a sterile clamp, which I put in place. Then he clamped the new plastic clamp in place, but there wasn't much room left to properly place the clamp. A tiny bit of the baby's skin was under the plastic clamp. I took the baby to the nursery, as was the usual practice at the time. I needed to call the pediatrician and of course, it was one with a reputation for being mean to nurses. I explained the situation to him, and I loved his reply.

"Well, you'll never do that again."

He was right. I never have. Each time I cut a cord; I am cautious to make sure I have cut it in the right place. Nothing else could have made me so particular about that one procedure.

Mistakes should be avoided, but if you do make one, learn from it.

TWENTY-THREE

BEING IN CHARGE

There are parts of the job that can only be learned by doing.

It will happen before you think it should. You will come in for your shift and *you* will be in charge. Most of the time, you will feel inadequate for the position. Almost everyone feels that way. Those who think they are ready usually aren't.

Before that day, there are some things you can do to help you feel prepared. Watch your charge nurse. How does she handle emergencies? How does she assign patients? Does the Charge Nurse assist with admissions and discharges? Ask questions regarding how and why they do what they do. If there are forms to be filled out during the shift, such as census and/or staffing sheets, ask if you can start filling them out. That way, when the time comes, you will feel more comfortable doing it.

However, some parts of the job can only be learned by doing it. When you begin being in charge you will have a greater appreciation for other Charge Nurses. The more often you are in charge, the more you will recognize which staff nurses are best for each task. You will also learn which physicians and ancillary staff require notification in different situations. You will understand who needs help with procedures and who does not. It will come with time.

Like the Nurse Manager, the Charge Nurse wears a heavy coat of responsibility. Not only are they in charge, but they frequently have patients as well.

Charge Nurses should know what is happening with all the patients under their care. Many prefer to help with admissions, so they are familiar with the patients on their unit. Charge Nurses should help when it is reasonable to do so.

They should also be present during any emergency. They may be called to make certain decisions or to communicate with the House Supervisor regarding special needs in a particular emergency.

Sometimes, as a Charge Nurse, you may have situations in which you honestly do not know what to do. If you reach this point, contact your House Supervisor. If that doesn't answer your question, contact your Nurse Manager. You always have someone you can call, even in the middle of the night.

One of the things that will be part of your job as a Charge Nurse may be correcting the nurses in your unit. The best way to do this is very gently. Remember, we were all new nurses once, and we have all made mistakes. Approach learning as a team and use established documentation to verify your instruction.

For instance, electronic fetal monitoring interpretation is often difficult for new Labor & Delivery nurses. There are clear-cut definitions for decreases in the baby's heartbeat, but tracings can still be hard to interpret. Discussing the established definitions while interpreting the tracing can help newer nurses learn systematic and effective ways to approach fetal monitor interpretation. The most important thing is to *maintain respect for the nurses*. Respecting them makes them feel more comfortable asking for help in the future. Being gentle and kind teaches more than the subject at hand. It also demonstrates to the young nurse how they should respond to others.

This is especially important since they may one day be Charge Nurses themselves

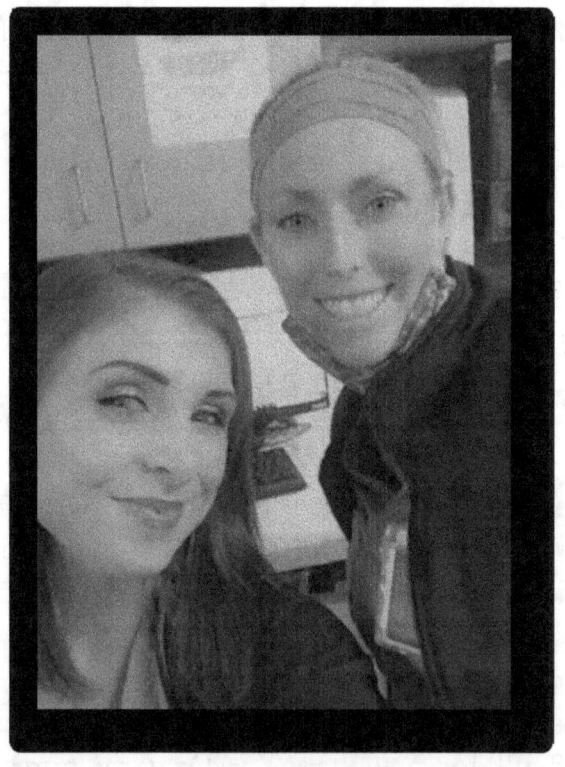

Ashlee and Jess

TWENTY-FOUR

THE PHYSICIANS

We are not required to like the physicians but to work with them professionally and respectfully.

In your nursing career, you will meet all types of physicians. Many physicians consider the nurse an essential collaborator in the care of the patient, which we are. They may ask your opinion and genuinely want to know what you think.

I had only been working in the NICU for a few months when a resident came to me and asked if one of my babies could tolerate coming off the ventilator. I turned around to see to whom he was talking. He said, "You are the one weighing and suctioning the baby. You know best what he can tolerate and can't." Having a physician ask my opinion – in the 1970's - was huge to me. I couldn't believe a physician valued my opinion! You may have this happen often in your career, which will be a token of their respect for you.

Some physicians may treat you poorly regardless of your knowledge base, skill level, and certification. Some may even criticize or make fun of you for no reason at all, though I notice less of that now than when began as a nurse. Hopefully, you will work with physicians who treat you with the respect you deserve.

Some may become your friends. How you approach this friendship in the hospital is important. You must maintain an attitude of respect, even if you socialize with the physician outside the hospital. Your behavior will be an example to others.

Many physicians love to teach, and you can learn much from them. Take advantage of their teaching and learn all you can.

If you have a valid issue with a physician, the best first step is to take it to your Nurse Manager. She is able to discuss the issue with the physician in ways that would be inappropriate for a staff nurse.

Try to maintain a professional, calm composure when dealing with a troublesome physician and if you must, just walk away.

TWENTY-FIVE

WHAT ABOUT LAWSUITS?

Don't talk. Don't talk. Don't talk.

Every nurse hates that word, *lawsuits*. Yes, lawsuits can happen, but less frequently than you think. There are, however, some things you need to understand about them.

Just because a lawsuit includes you does not mean you have done anything wrong or that you are not a good nurse. It is often customary for plaintiff's attorneys to subpoena every name they see on the chart in hopes someone may have a tidbit of information that may help their case. I even saw a court summons that named a person whose signature was illegible. The summons described them as "someone to be identified at a later date." We were asked later by the plaintiff's attorneys if we could decipher the signature. You could be named in the lawsuit to see if you can give information they haven't gotten from other sources.

If a lawsuit includes you, the institution you work in may have already met with you. There are things you need to know about the process and how you should – and shouldn't - respond to the lawsuit:

- -Most nurses assume if a lawsuit includes them, they are at risk of losing their license. That is not likely to happen unless you have committed gross negligence.
- -A medical malpractice suit is a long process. The plaintiff usually has two years to file a lawsuit after the incident. Even after that, the process is painfully slow, sometimes taking years.
- .-Don't talk to anyone about it except your attorney. Anyone with whom you discuss the incident, even other nurses, can be subpoenaed for that information. *Don't talk.*
- -Stay away from social media and your phone. Even if you refer to the situation or the lawsuit in vague terms, it could still be possible for a plaintiff's attorney to misconstrue things you have said. Their goal would be to represent you, your hospital, or other healthcare professionals in a bad light. Attorneys can, and do, subpoena the cell phones of the staff involved. The plaintiff's attorneys might use any messages you have sent against you, or others involved in the case. *Don't talk. Don't talk.*
- -Don't fall into despair. As the process goes on, something may come to light that may remove you from the case entirely.

I was once one of multiple doctors, nurses, and even laboratory personnel named in a frivolous lawsuit. It upset me so much I wanted to change professions. As it turned out, I made an off-handed comment to the paralegal that the Chief Resident asked me specifically to take care of this patient when I first came in for my shift. She asked me a couple of questions about the situation and asked me to sit and wait. That information showed the Chief Resident was aware of the situation before I arrived, and the chain of command instituted. As a result, the judge dismissed me from the case. A few weeks later, the judge dismissed the entire case.

Your attorneys will prepare you well. In another case, the defense attorneys took much time preparing us for depositions. They explained legal terminology we may not have been familiar with. They explained nurses always want to "explain what happened," which was not good. They reinforced that if we didn't remember something, all we had to say was, "I don't recall."

The mock deposition was a real learning experience. The attorney pretending to be the plaintiff's attorney was much harder on me than the actual plaintiff's attorney in the deposition. I felt very well prepared and left the deposition knowing I had done the best I could, not only for myself but for the institution as well. The judge dismissed this case before going to trial.

If a nurse you work with is part of a lawsuit, do not ask them anything about the case. Do give them encouragement and support in any way you can. It is one of the most stressful things a nurse can experience, especially when you know you have done nothing wrong.

Don't talk. Don't talk. Don't talk.

TWENTY-SIX

YOUR EDUCATION ISN'T OVER

Keep studying and keep learning.

Once you have finished your nursing program and have that diploma, you may feel your education days are over. Nothing could be further from the truth. Nursing is a process of continued education. Not just the CE you need to maintain your license, but the education required to keep up with the changes in your profession.

The amount that newborn care has changed since I worked in the NICU 45 years ago is phenomenal. Labor & Delivery has greatly changed since I started there in 1983 as well. As nurses, we will always be adapting to new protocols and policies and studying new drugs. It is our responsibility to learn all this new information and keep our knowledge base and skill levels current.

Then, there is the issue of structured education. If you have graduated with an ADN, I strongly advise, after you have some experience under your belt, to pursue your BSN. If you graduated with your BSN, I recommend pursuing your MSN. I am not suggesting you leave bedside nursing, but that you make all the options available to you that you can. If you have a BSN or MSN, doors will be open to you if you become interested in them.

The best Nursery nurse I have ever known has her MSN in nursing education. But her one love, and her most incredible talent, is taking care of newborns and their parents. Working with her for over three decades has been a great blessing. The greatest blessing, though, was that she was able to care for most of my grandchildren as newborns.

There are other areas of learning open to you as well. You can pursue certifications in your specialty.

For example, Labor & Delivery nurses can study for certifications in Inpatient Obstetrics, Electronic Fetal Monitoring, Inpatient Antepartum Nursing, High-Risk Obstetrics Nursing, Maternal Newborn Nursing, and more.

Each specialty has certification tests that add credentials to your learning and experience. Certifications are a way to prove you have a thorough knowledge of your specialty.

Keep studying and keep learning. Earn certifications, go to conferences, and take classes.

Become a source of information for your patients, their families, and your co-workers.

TWENTY-SEVEN

PREPARE FOR THE FUTURE

One day you will realize you only have a few years until you can retire. This is not the time to begin planning for your retirement.

As you begin your nursing career, retirement may be the last thing on your mind. After all, it is a LONG way away. But it will go by so very fast. One day you will realize you only have a few years until you can retire. This is not the time to begin planning for your retirement.

As soon as possible, begin contributing to a 401K or IRA (Individual Retirement Account) if your institution offers one. Many hospitals will match at least a percentage of the amount contributed to a 401K. If not, open your own retirement fund and begin a steady contribution. It will be tempting to save that money for vacations or items you haven't been able to afford until now, but your retirement fund needs to be high on your list of priorities.

Automatic withdrawals from your paycheck are almost painless and you will soon be able to see how the money adds up.

Long before your retirement date, begin reading and studying about insurance options for retirement. It is not as straightforward as you may think. Attend classes on retirement income, insurance, and Medicare. Many of these are offered free online. Make yourself as knowledgeable about your retirement as you were about your career.

When the time comes to plan your retirement party, you will be so glad you have planned for the end of your career at the beginning of it.

As soon as possible, begin saving and planning for your retirement.

TWENTY-EIGHT

SAFETY MEASURES

Every single time.

In this day and time most people will not drive their vehicle without wearing a seatbelt. In fact, some cars will not engage to drive until everyone is buckled up. Most of us don't even consider it an option. As nurses, this is the same attitude we should have regarding our safety measures for our patients.

One way to protect our patients is to be knowledgeable of the policies and procedures of our institution. You can't perform what you don't know.

Practicing our profession without utilizing our institution's safety measures should not be an option. For instance, scanning the patient's armband and then their medication is one such safety precaution. Would it be quicker just to hand the patient the medicine. Yes, of course. Is it more likely we could give the medication to the wrong patient? Or give the wrong medication? Absolutely.

In the same manner, scanning the patient's bracelet before giving blood, or when labeling drawn blood, protects our patients. It takes a few more minutes, but the safety it provides is worth every second.

In Labor & Delivery one of our safety measures is to check the mother's band against the baby's band when a baby is returned to the mother. It only takes a minute, and there is no way a nurse will hand a mother the wrong baby if she does this every single time.

Of course, there are emergency situations in which it simply will not be possible to implement some safety measures, and most scanning systems accommodate those situations. But they should by far be the exception, rather than the rule. In most cases, the nurse should know the safety measures put into place by their institution and use them every single time.

Every single time.

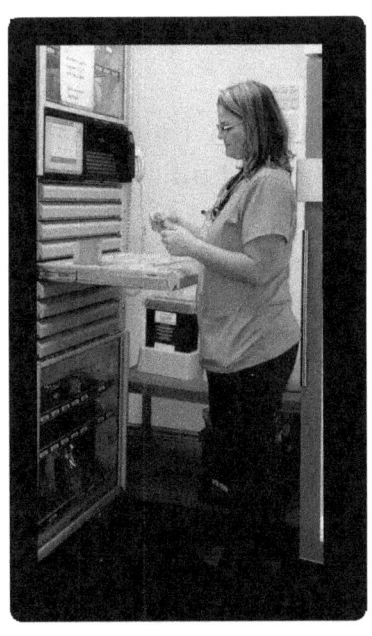

Coree double checking medication

TWENTY-NINE

DOWN-TIME

Keep the reminder that down-times do happen in the back of your mind and mentally prepare yourself for that possibility.

Periodically the computer systems in your institution will have down-time. The systems may be in the process of upgrading in which the down time usually lasts a short time. Or, as happened to my institution once, it could have been the victim of hacking. This meant charting on paper for weeks. Most of our nurses had never charted on paper, in fact they had never even seen the flowsheets we had used to chart prior to computerization. The older nurses sometimes found themselves dictating to the younger nurses exactly how to phrase their narrative assessments on paper.

One of the wonderful things about computerized charting is that the choices for what to chart are usually built into the screens. For example, if you are charting breath sounds, all the different types of breath sounds may be listed there for you to simply click on what is appropriate for that patient. But with paper charting, the different choices must come from your own head.

Sometimes when you are charting, look at all the different choices you see available. Are there any terms you don't recognize? When you have time, look them up. Think about how you would chart the assessment you just documented if you were charting on paper. What would you say? What order would you use to chart?

Keep the reminder that down-times do happen in the back of your mind and mentally prepare yourself for that possibility.

Prepare for down time before it happens.

THIRTY

DON'T TAKE IT PERSONAL

Try not to be offended.

There may be times when you begin your nursing career when more experienced nurses, and especially the Charge Nurse, may feel the need to check behind your assessments. Try not to be offended.

When I was first working as a newly graduated nurse, I worked for a few months in the Cardiac Care Unit. There were two or three of us "new grads" on the night shift. At the beginning of the shift, we would assess our patients and take their vital signs. It wasn't long after beginning to work in the unit, we realized the Charge Nurse was going behind us and assessing the patient and taking their vital signs as well. We were all offended at this. It wasn't until years later when I was a Charge Nurse with new nurses on my shift that I realized why she had done this. She felt personally responsible for *all* the patients in her unit, and she knew that not every new nurse had honed her skills to the level they need to be for a critical care unit. This was before the days of specific unit orientation programs or preceptor programs.

If another nurse checks behind you, or gives you advice about a particular procedure, skill or assessment, try to take it in stride. They are showing a desire for you to develop into the very best nurse you can be and are trying to assist you with that goal. They likely have expertise and tips to share with you which can be invaluable in your day-to-day working. Listen to them carefully and if you have any questions, this would be the proper time to vocalize them.

Remember, every experienced and "seasoned" nurse out there was once the new nurse on the unit.

We have all had to walk that path and learn from others.

THIRTY-ONE

ESSENTIAL KNOWLEDGE

*The Nurse Practice Act, Specialty Standards of Care,
and Institutional Policies and Procedures are our
foundation.*

Finally, I have saved what is the most important and undoubtedly the most boring for last.

All nurses must possess three essential pieces of knowledge. They serve as the heart of our profession. This information is not entertaining but vital to our practical nursing experience.

The first is the scope of the Nurse Practice Act for the state in which we practice. The second is the Standards of Care for our specialty, and the third is the Policies and Procedures for the institution where we work. It is our responsibility to read these, know them, and know how to access them.

The Nurse Practice Act is specific to each state. What is acceptable for an RN in California differs from that in

Alabama. We are each responsible for knowing what we can and cannot do in our state.

The Standards of Care for our specialty outline expected actions in a specific order for routine and critical situations. These are usually in the form of protocols. Each nurse must know these and mentally prepare herself to perform them without having to stop and think or ask questions. We are each also expected to know where to find them if asked.

The third is the Policies, Procedures, and Protocols of the institution where we work. These govern our actions daily and are usually voted upon by a committee of physicians who practice the associated specialty at that institution. Even if the Nurse Practice Act in a specific state gives authority to nurses to perform a particular procedure, if the institution in which she works doesn't, she should not be doing that procedure.

We must not rely on others working with us to provide information contained in our Policies and Procedures. Asking someone else is different than knowing how to find the information. Some people may give incomplete, out-of-date, or simply wrong information. We should be able to access our facility's Policies and Procedures anytime.

Once, I watched a fetal monitor strip with a physician. She asked about the patient's Pitocin rate.

I told her, and she said, "Well, turn it up."

I explained the patient was consistently having more than five contractions in ten minutes, so the rate could not be increased.

"Of course, it can. I'm the doctor and giving the order, so you have to do it," was her reply.

Without questioning someone else or looking it up, I told her, "No, increasing the Pitocin if a patient consistently has more than five contractions in ten minutes is against the Pitocin Protocol."

I also told her the protocols protect the patient, and the hospital paid me to follow those protocols. While she was unhappy about it then, she later realized I was correct.

Our foundation is the Nurse Practice Act, Specialty Standards of Care, and Institutional Policies and Procedures. They support and protect our patients, and they support, and protect us. Whenever we step outside any of these, we put our patients - and ourselves- in dangerous positions. If we read nothing else about our profession, we must read these.

Knowing what to do in a complicated case is one thing, which is the "what." But we must also know the "why." Understanding the reasoning behind the actions makes all the difference in patient care.

For example, an obstetric patient on Magnesium needs her urine output measured hourly. Why? Magnesium is excreted in the urine. If the patient's urine output is insufficient, their magnesium blood levels will be higher. Knowing this explains why we do the "what," in this case, checking urine output every hour.

If there is a standard of care you need help understanding, ask for the "why". It will help you understand and remember the "what". If your preceptor can't give you a clear explanation, ask your nurse manager. Review the policies and procedures and the Standards of Care. These often explain not only the processes, but the rationale for them.

Understanding the *why* is the key to properly performing the *what*.

CONCLUSION

Nursing is an incredible profession. It is hard work, but it is also very gratifying.

Much of doing it well is common sense.

Be thankful nurses no longer wear those white hats!

Do the right thing because it is the right thing to do.

Don't loan your favorite pen to anyone, especially a physician!

If you don't know the answer, look it up. Sometimes, you will get an incorrect answer by asking someone.

Listen to that little voice inside of you. It is rarely wrong.

Don't be embarrassed to make lists of what you need to do each shift.

Spend money on good shoes.

A good Care Tech is worth their weight in gold.

Be kind. Be thoughtful. Be respectful to your patients, visitors, the physicians, and the staff.

Clean up after yourself. Don't leave a patient's room a mess.

Invest in a good stethoscope.

Keep an extra set of underwear and a can of soup in your locket. One day they might come in handy.

Caring for others is a great privilege and a great responsibility. Never take it for granted.

Treat your patients as you would want someone to treat your loved ones.

Hold a patient's hand. Wipe their forehead. Feed them some ice cubes. Sometimes, just sitting by a patient and listening is the best gift you can give them.

Enjoy your career.

You will make great friends. You will share much laughter, share some tears, share your lunch, and maybe even share that favorite pen. It will go by so fast, and before you know it, your retirement will begin. Enjoy that, too. You will have earned it!

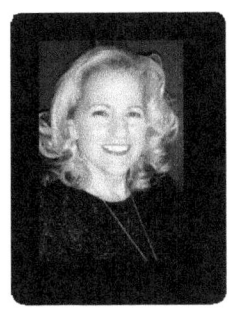

ABOUT THE AUTHOR

Frances Davis has been a Registered Nurse for over 45 years. She has worked in NICU, Mother-Baby, and Labor and Delivery. During fourteen of her 36 years as a Labor & Delivery nurse, she was the Assistant Manager of her unit.

At the request of her hospital, she spent three years as a Clinical Analyst on the Information Technology team to build, teach and implement computerized charting.

She has been an instructor for Community Education, Childbirth Education, Infant CPR, Newborn Care, Early Pregnancy Classes, Facts of Life classes for young girls and yearly Unit Competencies for Labor & Delivery.

She has been in over 4,000 deliveries and delivered nearly 100 babies herself.

She loves mothers and babies and has had an enjoyable career caring for them. This book is her way of giving back to a profession that has given so much to her.

"This is the Lord's doing, and it is marvelous in our eyes."
Psalm 118:23

www.ingramcontent.com/pod-product-compliance
Lightning Source LLC
Chambersburg PA
CBHW071158290526
45796CB00007B/72